Exercise & Gout

How to Stay Active

HR Research Alliance

Disclaimer

The information provided in this book is intended for general informational purposes only and is not a substitute for professional medical advice, diagnosis, or treatment. The content is based on personal experiences, research, and expert opinions, but it should not be considered a comprehensive guide for managing gout or any other medical condition.

Readers are strongly encouraged to consult with their healthcare providers before starting any new exercise program, making dietary changes, or using any nutritional supplements. Individual health conditions and needs can vary greatly, and only a qualified healthcare professional can provide personalized advice and treatment.

Introduction

This book is designed to be your comprehensive guide to managing gout through exercise, providing you with the knowledge, tools, and motivation to lead a more active and healthier life despite the challenges of joint pain.

Purpose of the Book

Gout, a form of arthritis characterized by sudden and severe pain in the joints, can be a debilitating condition. Many people believe that physical activity is off-limits when dealing with such pain. However, research shows that staying active is not only possible but also beneficial for managing gout. The purpose of this book is to:

- **Educate:** Provide a thorough understanding of what gout is, its causes, and how it affects the body.

- **Empower:** Equip you with safe and effective exercise routines tailored for individuals with gout.

- **Encourage:** Offer motivational insights and real-life success stories to inspire you on your journey to better health.

Understanding Gout and the Importance of Exercise

Gout is caused by the accumulation of uric acid crystals in the joints, leading to intense pain, inflammation, and swelling. While it may seem counterintuitive, exercise plays a crucial role in managing gout. Regular physical activity helps:

- **Reduce inflammation:** Exercise can help lower uric acid levels and reduce inflammation, thereby decreasing the frequency and severity of gout attacks.

- **Improve joint function:** Strengthening muscles around the joints can provide better support and stability, reducing pain and improving mobility.

- **Enhance overall health:** Staying active boosts cardiovascular health, aids in weight management, and improves mental well-being, all of which are important for managing gout.

Motivational Message to Inspire Readers

Living with gout can be challenging, but it does not have to define your life. Every step you take, no matter how small, is a victory. This book is not just about providing information; it's about empowering you to take control of your health and live your life to the fullest. Remember, the journey to managing gout through exercise is a marathon, not a sprint. Celebrate your progress, be patient with yourself, and keep moving forward. You have the strength to overcome the challenges of gout and achieve a healthier, more active lifestyle.

Understanding Gout

What is Gout?

Definition and Causes

Gout is a type of arthritis that occurs when there is an excess of uric acid in the blood, leading to the formation of sharp, needle-like crystals in the joints and surrounding tissues. These crystals cause sudden, severe episodes of pain, tenderness, redness, warmth, and swelling, often in the big toe, but they can also affect other joints such as the ankles, knees, elbows, wrists, and fingers.

Primary causes:

- **Hyperuricemia**: High levels of uric acid in the blood, often due to the body's inability to efficiently eliminate uric acid through the kidneys.

- **Genetic factors:** A family history of gout increases the likelihood of developing the condition.

- **Diet:** High intake of purine-rich foods (e.g., red meat, seafood), sugary beverages, and alcohol can elevate uric acid levels.

Symptoms and Diagnosis

Gout symptoms can develop quickly, often occurring at night, and can last for days or weeks.

Symptoms:

- Intense joint pain

- Swelling and redness

- Heat and tenderness in the affected area

- Limited range of motion in the affected joint

Diagnosis:

- **Medical history and physical examination:** Assessing the patient's symptoms and family history of gout.

- **Joint fluid test:** Extracting fluid from the affected joint to look for urate crystals under a microscope.

- **Blood test:** Measuring the levels of uric acid in the blood.

- **Imaging tests:** X-rays, ultrasound, or dual-energy CT scans to detect urate crystals in joints.

The Role of Uric Acid

How It Affects Joints

Uric acid is a waste product formed from the breakdown of purines, which are substances found naturally in the body and in certain foods.

Normally, uric acid dissolves in the blood and passes through the kidneys into the urine. However, when the body produces too much uric acid or the kidneys excrete too little, uric acid can build up, forming sharp, needle-like crystals in a joint or surrounding tissue that cause pain, inflammation, and swelling.

Triggers for Gout Attacks

Several factors can trigger gout attacks:

- **Dietary choices:** Consuming large amounts of purine-rich foods, alcohol, and sugary drinks.

- **Medications:** Certain drugs like diuretics, aspirin, and immunosuppressants can increase uric acid levels.

- **Health conditions:** Obesity, hypertension, diabetes, and kidney disease.

- **Dehydration:** Insufficient fluid intake can increase uric acid concentration.

- **Stress and trauma:** Physical or emotional stress, and injuries to the joints.

Common Myths and Facts

Debunking Misconceptions

1. Myth: Gout is solely caused by poor dietary choices.

Fact: While diet plays a role, genetics and other health conditions are significant factors.

2. Myth: Only older men get gout.

Fact: Gout can affect people of all ages and genders, although it is more common in middle-aged men and postmenopausal women.

3. Myth: Gout is a rare condition.

Fact: Gout is relatively common, affecting millions of people worldwide.

Scientific Evidence and Findings

Scientific research continues to shed light on gout, improving our understanding and management of the condition:

- **Genetic studies:** Identifying genes that influence uric acid metabolism.

- **Dietary studies:** Investigating the impact of specific foods and dietary patterns on uric acid levels.

- **Medication advancements:** Developing new treatments to reduce uric acid levels and prevent gout attacks.

- **Lifestyle research:** Exploring the benefits of exercise, weight management, and stress reduction in managing gout.

By dispelling myths and providing accurate information, this chapter aims to build a solid foundation of knowledge about gout, helping readers better understand their condition and how to manage it effectively.

The Importance of Staying Active

Benefits of Exercise for Gout Sufferers

Reducing Inflammation and Pain

Regular exercise can help manage gout by reducing inflammation and pain in several ways:

- **Anti-inflammatory effects:** Physical activity can decrease levels of inflammatory markers in the body, helping to control the inflammatory response associated with gout.

- **Pain relief:** Exercise stimulates the release of endorphins, the body's natural painkillers, which can help alleviate gout pain.

Improving Joint Function and Flexibility

Exercise plays a crucial role in maintaining and enhancing joint health, particularly for those with gout:

- **Increased range of motion:** Regular movement helps to maintain and improve the range of motion in affected joints, preventing stiffness and improving flexibility.

- **Strengthening muscles:** Building muscle around joints can provide better support and reduce the strain on joints, leading to less pain and improved function.

- **Joint lubrication:** Movement helps distribute synovial fluid, which nourishes and lubricates the joints, reducing friction and pain.

Enhancing Overall Health and Well-being

The benefits of exercise extend beyond joint health to overall physical well-being:

- **Weight management:** Regular exercise helps to control body weight, reducing the stress on joints and lowering uric acid levels.

- **Cardiovascular health:** Exercise improves heart health, reducing the risk of cardiovascular diseases often associated with gout.

- **Metabolic health:** Physical activity can enhance insulin sensitivity and glucose metabolism, which is beneficial for those with gout who also have metabolic syndrome or diabetes.

Mental Health Benefits

Reducing Stress and Anxiety

Managing stress and anxiety is crucial for gout sufferers, as these factors can trigger gout flares:

- **Stress reduction:** Exercise helps to reduce levels of stress hormones like cortisol, promoting a sense of calm and relaxation.

- **Anxiety management:** Regular physical activity can decrease symptoms of anxiety, providing a natural outlet for releasing pent-up tension.

Boosting Mood and Mental Resilience

The positive impact of exercise on mental health can be significant:

- **Mood enhancement:** Exercise stimulates the production of neurotransmitters like serotonin and dopamine, which are essential for mood regulation and can help alleviate feelings of depression.

- **Mental resilience:** Engaging in regular physical activity can enhance mental resilience, helping individuals cope better with the challenges of living with a chronic condition like gout.

- **Self-esteem and confidence:** Achieving fitness goals and maintaining an active lifestyle can boost self-esteem and confidence, contributing to a more positive outlook on life.

By highlighting the multifaceted benefits of exercise, this chapter aims to inspire readers to incorporate physical activity into their daily routine, not only to manage gout symptoms but also to improve their overall quality of life. Through regular exercise, gout sufferers can experience a range of physical and mental health benefits that contribute to better management of their condition and enhanced well-being.

Preparing for Exercise

Consulting with Healthcare Providers

Importance of Professional Guidance

- **Personalized Advice:** Gout affects each individual differently, so it's crucial to get tailored advice from healthcare providers who understand your specific condition.

- **Safety First:** Professionals can identify any contraindications to exercise and suggest modifications to ensure you exercise safely.

- **Integrated Approach:** Working with doctors, physical therapists, and possibly dietitians can provide a holistic approach to managing gout alongside exercise.

Tailoring Exercise Plans to Individual Needs

- **Assessment of Condition:** A thorough assessment of your gout condition, including the frequency and severity of flare-ups, helps in creating a customized exercise plan.

- **Exercise Prescription:** Professionals can recommend specific exercises that benefit gout sufferers, focusing on low-impact activities that minimize joint stress.

- **Adjustments Over Time:** Regular consultations allow for adjustments to the exercise plan based on your progress and any changes in your condition.

Setting Realistic Goals

Creating Achievable Fitness Milestones

- **SMART Goals:** Set Specific, Measurable, Achievable, Relevant, and Time-bound goals to guide your fitness journey.

- **Incremental Progress:** Start with small, manageable activities and gradually increase intensity and duration to avoid overexertion.

- **Short-term vs. Long-term Goals:** Define both short-term and long-term goals to keep motivation high and maintain a sense of direction.

Tracking Progress and Celebrating Success

- **Monitoring Tools:** Use tools like fitness apps, journals, or wearable devices to track your exercise routines, progress, and any changes in symptoms.

- **Regular Reviews:** Periodically review your progress with your healthcare provider to ensure you are on the right track.

- **Celebrating Milestones:** Acknowledge and celebrate your achievements, no matter how small, to stay motivated and positive.

Safety Precautions

Recognizing Signs of Overexertion

- **Understanding Limits:** Learn to listen to your body and recognize signs of overexertion, such as excessive fatigue, prolonged soreness, or joint pain.

- **Rest and Recovery:** Incorporate rest days into your exercise routine to allow your body to recover and prevent overtraining.

- **Hydration and Nutrition:** Maintain proper hydration and nutrition to support your exercise efforts and overall health.

Managing Flare-ups and Preventing Injury

- **Flare-up Management:** Have a plan in place for managing flare-ups, including rest, medication, and modifications to your exercise routine.

- **Warm-up and Cool-down:** Always include proper warm-up and cool-down exercises to prepare your body for activity and aid in recovery.

- **Low-impact Activities:** Focus on low-impact exercises like swimming, cycling, or walking, which are gentler on the joints.

- **Proper Technique:** Ensure you use proper techniques and postures during exercise to avoid unnecessary strain or injury. By carefully preparing for exercise, gout sufferers can maximize the benefits of physical activity while minimizing the risk of injury or flare-ups.

Types of Exercises for Gout Management

Low-Impact Aerobic Exercises

Walking

Benefits

- **Joint-Friendly:** Walking is a low-impact exercise that minimizes stress on the joints, making it ideal for gout sufferers.

- **Cardiovascular Health:** Regular walking improves cardiovascular health, reducing the risk of heart disease.

- **Weight Management:** Helps in maintaining a healthy weight, which can reduce the frequency and severity of gout flare-ups.

Tips for Starting

- **Start Slow:** Begin with short walks and gradually increase the duration and intensity.

- **Proper Footwear:** Invest in comfortable, supportive shoes to prevent foot and joint pain.

- **Consistency:** Aim for a regular walking schedule, such as 30 minutes a day, five days a week.

Swimming

Benefits

- **Full-Body Workout:** Swimming engages multiple muscle groups, providing a comprehensive workout.

- **Buoyancy:** Water buoyancy reduces the impact on joints, making it an excellent option for those with joint pain.

- **Flexibility and Strength:** Improves flexibility and strengthens muscles without causing strain.

Tips for Starting

- **Find a Pool:** Look for a local pool with lap swimming or a fitness gym with water aerobics classes.

- **Warm-Up:** Perform gentle stretches before entering the pool to prepare your muscles.

- **Begin with Basics:** Start with simple strokes like freestyle, side stroke, or backstroke, and gradually try more complex techniques if desired, but not necessary.

Cycling

Benefits

- **Low-Impact:** Cycling is gentle on the joints while providing an effective cardiovascular workout.

- **Muscle Strengthening:** Strengthens the lower body muscles, including the legs, hips, and glutes.

- **Adaptability:** Can be done indoors on a stationary bike or outdoors, offering flexibility in your exercise routine.

Tips for Starting

- **Adjust the Bike:** Ensure your bike is properly adjusted to your height to avoid strain on your knees and back.

- **Gradual Progression:** Start with short, easy rides and gradually increase the duration and intensity.

- **Safety Gear:** Wear appropriate safety gear, including a helmet and reflective clothing if cycling outdoors.

By incorporating these low-impact aerobic exercises into their routines, gout sufferers can enjoy the numerous benefits of regular physical activity while minimizing the risk of exacerbating their symptoms.

Walking, swimming, and cycling provide accessible and effective ways to stay active and improve overall health.

Strength Training

Importance of Muscle Strengthening

- **Joint Support:** Strengthening the muscles around affected joints can provide better support and stability, potentially reducing pain and the frequency of gout attacks.

- **Improved Functionality:** Enhanced muscle strength can improve overall mobility and functionality, making daily activities easier and less painful.

- **Reduced Risk of Injury:** Stronger muscles can help prevent injuries by supporting joints more effectively and reducing the likelihood of falls or strains.

Safe Weight Training Techniques

Start with Light Weights

- **Beginner-Friendly:** Start with lighter weights to learn proper form and technique without putting excessive strain on the joints.

- **Gradual Increase:** Slowly increase the weight as your strength improves to avoid overloading the joints.

Focus on Form

- **Proper Technique:** Emphasize correct form and technique to avoid injury and maximize the effectiveness of the exercises.

- **Controlled Movements:** Perform exercises with controlled, steady movements to reduce the risk of joint stress.

Use Low-Impact Equipment

- **Resistance Bands:** These provide resistance without heavy weights, allowing for effective strength training with minimal impact on the joints.

- **Bodyweight Exercises:** Utilize exercises like squats, lunges, and push-ups that use your body weight for resistance and require no additional equipment.

Incorporate Full-Body Workouts

- **Balanced Routine:** Focus on a balanced workout that includes exercises for all major muscle groups to ensure overall strength and stability.

- **Functional Movements:** Include functional movements that mimic daily activities, helping to improve practical strength and endurance.

Allow for Rest and Recovery

- **Rest Days:** Ensure you have adequate rest between strength training sessions to allow muscles and joints to recover.

- **Listen to Your Body:** Pay attention to any signs of discomfort or pain and adjust your workout accordingly to prevent overuse injuries.

Seek Professional Guidance

- **Consult a Trainer:** Consider working with a certified trainer who has experience working with individuals with joint issues to create a safe and effective strength training program.

- **Medical Advice:** Always consult with your healthcare provider before starting any new exercise regimen, especially if you have specific health concerns related to gout.

By integrating strength training into their exercise routines, individuals with gout can build muscle strength and improve joint support while minimizing the risk of injury. Emphasizing proper technique, starting with light weights, and incorporating low-impact equipment can help ensure that strength training remains a safe and beneficial part of managing gout.

Flexibility and Stretching

Yoga and Pilates for Joint Health

Yoga

- **Gentle Movements:** Yoga incorporates gentle, controlled movements that can improve flexibility, balance, and joint health without putting excessive strain on the body.

- **Variety of Poses:** Focus on poses that enhance joint mobility and strengthen surrounding muscles, such as child's pose, cat-cow, and gentle twists.

- **Breathing Techniques:** Yoga encourages deep breathing, which can help with relaxation and reduce stress, potentially lessening the frequency of gout attacks.

- **Modifications:** Use props such as blocks and straps to modify poses and accommodate any limitations caused by gout.

Pilates

- **Core Strength:** Pilates focuses on strengthening the core muscles, which can help stabilize the body and improve overall posture and alignment, benefiting joint health.

- **Low-Impact Movements**: Pilates exercises are typically low-impact and can be adapted to avoid stressing affected joints.

- **Controlled Exercises**: Emphasize precise, controlled movements to enhance flexibility and strength without causing excessive strain.

Simple Stretching Routines

Morning Stretching Routine

- **Gentle Warm-Up**: Start with a gentle warm-up, such as marching in place or light walking, to prepare the muscles and joints for stretching.

- **Key Stretches**: Incorporate stretches targeting common problem areas such as the calves, hamstrings, quadriceps, and hips. Examples include calf stretches, hamstring stretches, and hip flexor stretches.

- **Hold and Breathe:** Hold each stretch for 15-30 seconds and focus on deep, steady breathing to help relax the muscles and improve flexibility.

Evening Stretching Routine

- **Relaxation Focus:** Include stretches that promote relaxation and prepare the body for rest, such as forward bends, seated stretches, and gentle twists.

- **Comfortable Positions:** Perform stretches while seated or lying down to reduce pressure on the joints and ensure comfort.

- **Consistency:** Aim to stretch daily or several times a week to maintain flexibility and prevent stiffness.

Stretching Tips

- **Warm Up First:** Always warm up the body with light activity before stretching to avoid injury and improve the effectiveness of the stretches.

- **Listen to Your Body:** Stretch only to the point of mild tension and avoid any movements that cause pain or discomfort.

- **Regular Practice:** Consistency is key to improving flexibility and maintaining joint health. Incorporate stretching into your regular exercise routine for the best results.

Integrating flexibility and stretching exercises into your routine can significantly benefit individuals with gout by improving joint mobility, reducing stiffness, and enhancing overall comfort.

Whether through yoga, Pilates, or simple stretching routines, maintaining a regular practice can help manage symptoms and promote a more active, pain-free lifestyle.

Creating an Exercise Routine

Designing a Balanced Plan

Combining Different Types of Exercises

- **Incorporate Variety:** A well-rounded exercise routine should include a mix of aerobic, strength, and flexibility exercises to address different aspects of fitness and support overall joint health.

- **Aerobic Exercise:** Activities such as walking, swimming, or cycling improve cardiovascular health and help manage weight, which can reduce stress on joints.

- **Strength Training:** Incorporate resistance exercises to build muscle strength and support joint stability. Focus on major muscle groups and use bodyweight or light weights.

- **Flexibility Training:** Include stretching and flexibility exercises like yoga or Pilates to enhance range of motion and prevent stiffness.

Structuring Weekly Workout Schedules

- **Weekly Breakdown:** Aim for a balanced weekly schedule that includes various types of exercises:

  - **Aerobic:** 3-4 days per week, with 30-45 minutes of moderate-intensity activity.

  - **Strength Training:** 2-3 days per week, allowing rest days in between to recover muscles.

  - **Flexibility:** Incorporate daily or every-other-day stretching or flexibility exercises.

- **Rest and Recovery:** Include at least one full rest day per week to allow the body to recover. Adjust the schedule based on individual needs and how the body responds.

Adapting to Individual Needs

Modifying Exercises for Different Fitness Levels

- **Start Slow:** Begin with low-intensity exercises and gradually increase intensity as fitness improves. Modify exercises to match current fitness levels and avoid overexertion.

- **Use Modifications:** Adjust exercises to accommodate limitations. For example, perform seated exercises if standing is uncomfortable or use resistance bands for lighter resistance.

- **Progress Gradually:** Increase the duration, intensity, or frequency of exercises gradually to prevent injury and allow the body to adapt.

Considering Comorbid Conditions

- **Understand Limitations:** If you have additional health conditions such as arthritis, diabetes, or cardiovascular issues, tailor the exercise plan to manage these conditions safely.

- **Consult Healthcare Providers:** Work with healthcare providers to create a comprehensive exercise plan that considers all health conditions and ensures safety.

- **Adjust as Needed:** Be prepared to adjust the routine based on how other conditions affect your ability to exercise.

Staying Consistent and Motivated

Overcoming Barriers to Exercise

- **Identify Barriers:** Common barriers include lack of time, pain, or motivation. Identify personal obstacles and develop strategies to address them.

- **Create a Routine:** Establish a consistent exercise routine by scheduling workouts at convenient times and making them a priority.

- **Start Small:** Begin with short, manageable workouts and gradually increase duration and intensity to build confidence and establish a habit.

Finding Support and Accountability

- **Social Support:** Engage friends, family, or exercise groups for motivation and encouragement. Share your goals with others to create a support network.

- **Professional Guidance:** Consider working with a personal trainer or physical therapist, especially one with experience in managing gout, to receive personalized guidance and support.

- **Track Progress:** Use a journal or fitness app to track workouts, set goals, and monitor progress. Celebrate achievements, no matter how small, to stay motivated.

Creating a tailored exercise routine that balances different types of exercises and adapts to individual needs is crucial for managing gout effectively. By designing a balanced plan, adjusting for personal limitations and comorbid conditions, and staying consistent and motivated, individuals with gout can maintain an active lifestyle and improve overall health and well-being.

Nutrition and Hydration

Dietary Considerations for Gout

Foods to Avoid and Include

Foods to Avoid:

- **High-Purine Foods:** Limit intake of foods high in purines, which can increase uric acid levels. These include red meats, organ meats (like liver), and certain types of seafood (such as sardines and anchovies).

- **Sugary Foods and Beverages:** Reduce consumption of sugary foods and beverages, particularly those high in fructose, as they can contribute to increased uric acid levels and exacerbate gout symptoms.

- **Alcohol:** Limit or avoid alcohol, particularly beer and spirits, as they can increase uric acid production and interfere with its excretion.

Foods to Include:

- **Low-Purine Foods:** Emphasize low-purine foods, such as fruits, vegetables, whole grains, and low-fat dairy products.

- **Anti-Inflammatory Foods:** Incorporate foods with anti-inflammatory properties, such as fatty fish (like salmon), nuts, seeds, and foods rich in antioxidants (such as berries).

- **Cherries and Berries:** Cherries, strawberries, and blueberries have been shown to help reduce uric acid levels and inflammation.

Importance of Hydration

- **Adequate Water Intake:** Drinking plenty of water helps to flush uric acid from the body and can reduce the risk of gout attacks. Aim for at least 8-10 glasses of water per day.

- **Limit Dehydrating Beverages:** Reduce the intake of beverages that can dehydrate the body, such as caffeinated drinks and alcohol. Choose water or herbal teas as primary fluids.

Nutritional Supplements

Potential Benefits and Risks

Common Supplements:

- **Vitamin C:** May help lower uric acid levels. Consult with a healthcare provider before starting a new supplement regimen.

- **Omega-3 Fatty Acids:** Found in fish oil supplements, may help reduce inflammation and joint pain.

- **Cherry Extract:** Some studies suggest that cherry extract can help lower uric acid levels and reduce the frequency of gout attacks.

Risks and Considerations:

- **Dosage and Purity:** Ensure supplements are taken in appropriate doses and are of high quality to avoid potential adverse effects.

- **Interactions:** Be aware of potential interactions between supplements and medications. Always consult with a healthcare provider before starting any new supplements.

Consulting with Healthcare Providers

- **Professional Guidance:** Work with a healthcare provider or registered dietitian to develop a nutrition plan tailored to individual needs and health conditions.

- **Regular Monitoring:** Regularly monitor uric acid levels and adjust dietary and supplement choices as needed based on professional advice.

- **Personalized Advice:** Seek personalized advice to address specific dietary needs and ensure that any supplements are appropriate for your health condition and overall well-being.

Proper nutrition and hydration play a crucial role in managing gout and supporting an active lifestyle. By making informed dietary choices, staying hydrated, and considering nutritional supplements with professional guidance, individuals with gout can better manage their condition and enhance their overall health.

Managing Gout Flare-Ups

Recognizing Early Signs

Identifying Triggers and Symptoms

Common Triggers:

 - **Dietary Factors:** Foods high in purines, excessive alcohol, and sugary beverages can trigger flare-ups.

 - **Stress and Illness:** Emotional stress, illness, or physical trauma can precipitate gout attacks.

 - **Medication Changes:** Adjustments in medications or non-compliance with prescribed treatments may trigger flare-ups.

Early Symptoms:

 - **Joint Pain:** Sudden, intense pain in the affected joint, often starting at night.

- **Redness and Swelling:** The joint may appear red, swollen, and feel warm to the touch.

- **Reduced Range of Motion:** Difficulty moving the affected joint due to pain and swelling.

Immediate Steps to Take

- **Rest the Affected Joint:** Minimize use of the affected joint to reduce stress and pain.

- **Apply Ice:** Use an ice pack wrapped in a cloth to apply cold to the joint for 15-20 minutes several times a day to reduce swelling and pain.

- **Elevate the Joint:** Elevate the affected joint to help reduce swelling.

- **Over-the-Counter Medications:** Consider over-the-counter anti-inflammatory medications like ibuprofen, following package instructions or advice from a healthcare provider.

Adjusting Exercise During Flare-Ups

Safe Activities and Modifications

- **Low-Impact Exercises:** Engage in low-impact activities that do not stress the affected joint, such as swimming or using an exercise bike.

- **Gentle Stretching:** Perform gentle stretching exercises to maintain flexibility without exacerbating pain.

- **Avoid High-Impact Activities:** Refrain from high-impact exercises or activities that put significant stress on the affected joint.

Rest and Recovery Strategies

- **Proper Rest:** Allow the joint ample time to rest and heal, avoiding activities that may provoke further pain.

- **Gradual Return to Exercise:** Once the flare-up subsides, gradually return to your regular exercise routine, starting with low-impact exercises and progressively increasing intensity.

- **Consultation with a Healthcare Provider:** Seek advice on when and how to resume exercise safely and adjust your exercise plan as needed.

Long-Term Management Strategies

Preventing Future Attacks

- **Maintain a Healthy Diet:** Adhere to a diet that minimizes purine intake and supports overall joint health.

- **Stay Hydrated:** Ensure adequate water intake to help prevent uric acid buildup.

- **Regular Exercise:** Consistently engage in low-impact exercises to maintain joint function and overall health.

Integrating Lifestyle Changes

- **Weight Management:** Achieve and maintain a healthy weight to reduce stress on joints and decrease the risk of gout attacks.

- **Stress Reduction:** Implement stress management techniques such as mindfulness, meditation, or relaxation exercises.

- **Routine Monitoring:** Regularly monitor uric acid levels and follow up with healthcare providers to adjust treatment and lifestyle changes as needed.

Effective management of gout flare-ups involves recognizing early symptoms, making temporary adjustments to exercise, and integrating long-term strategies for prevention. By staying informed and proactive, individuals with gout can better control their condition and maintain a more active and fulfilling lifestyle.

Real-Life Success Stories

Inspiring Stories of Gout Sufferers

Personal Journeys and Achievements

Case Study 1: John's Transformation:

- **Background:** John, diagnosed with gout in his 30s, faced severe pain that limited his daily activities.

- **Journey:** Through a combination of dietary changes, a tailored exercise plan, and regular medical consultations, John managed to significantly reduce his flare-ups and improve his quality of life.

- **Achievements:** John was able to participate in recreational activities he once thought impossible, such as hiking and playing sports with his children.

Case Study 2: Maria's Empowerment:

- **Background:** Maria struggled with frequent gout attacks that impacted her ability to work and enjoy her hobbies.

- **Journey:** By working closely with her healthcare provider and following a structured exercise routine along with dietary modifications, Maria experienced fewer flare-ups and regained her independence.

- **Achievements:** Maria successfully completed a half-marathon, a goal she had set before her diagnosis.

Case Study 3: Ahmed's Resilience:

- **Background:** Ahmed was diagnosed with gout in his late 40s and had to adapt his active lifestyle.

- **Journey:** Ahmed focused on low-impact exercises and embraced flexibility training to accommodate his condition.

- **Achievements:** Ahmed not only managed his symptoms but also became an advocate for others with gout, sharing his story and strategies through local support groups.

Overcoming Challenges and Setbacks

Facing Plateaus:

- **Challenge:** Many individuals encounter plateaus where progress seems to stall.

- **Solution:** Adapting exercise routines and re-evaluating dietary choices can help break through these plateaus. Seeking professional guidance can also provide new strategies for continued improvement.

Managing Unexpected Flare-Ups:

- **Challenge:** Flare-ups can occur unexpectedly and disrupt progress.

- **Solution:** Implementing a flexible exercise plan and having a proactive management strategy in place can help minimize the impact of flare-ups on overall progress.

Balancing Exercise with Daily Life:

- **Challenge:** Finding time to exercise while managing work, family, and other responsibilities can be difficult.

- **Solution:** Incorporating short, effective workouts into daily routines and setting realistic goals can make it easier to balance exercise with other life commitments.

Tips and Advice from the Community

Practical Advice from Fellow Sufferers

Start Slow and Build Gradually:

- **Tip:** Begin with low-impact exercises and gradually increase intensity to avoid overexertion.

- **Example:** Incorporate short walks or gentle stretches into your daily routine and gradually increase the duration and intensity as your body adapts.

Stay Hydrated and Mindful of Diet:

- **Tip:** Drink plenty of water and be mindful of dietary choices to manage uric acid levels effectively.

- **Example:** Aim for a balanced diet with low purine content and keep track of foods that may trigger flare-ups.

Listen to Your Body:

- **Tip:** Pay attention to how your body responds to different exercises and adjust accordingly.

- **Example:** If a particular activity causes discomfort, modify the exercise or choose an alternative that is better tolerated.

Building a Supportive Network

Join Support Groups:

- **Advice:** Connect with others who have gout to share experiences, advice, and encouragement.

- **Example:** Online forums, local support groups, or social media communities can provide valuable support and information.

Seek Professional Guidance:

- **Advice:** Regularly consult with healthcare providers, including dietitians and physical therapists, to stay informed and receive personalized advice.

- **Example:** Work with a dietitian to create a customized meal plan and a physical therapist to design an exercise routine tailored to your needs.

Share Your Journey:

- **Advice:** Share your experiences and progress with others to inspire and motivate both yourself and those around you.

- **Example:** Write a blog, participate in community events, or join online discussion groups to share your successes and challenges.

By highlighting real-life success stories and offering practical advice, this chapter aims to provide inspiration and actionable tips for facing similar challenges with gout. These uplifting stories and insights emphasize that managing gout effectively and staying active is achievable with the right strategies and support.

Advanced Strategies and Techniques

Innovative Exercise Methods

Latest Research and Trends

High-Intensity Interval Training (HIIT) and Gout:

- **Overview:** Research on the impact of HIIT on joint health and its suitability for gout sufferers.

- **Benefits:** Potential for improved cardiovascular health and metabolism without excessive strain on joints.

- **Considerations:** Guidelines for adapting HIIT workouts to suit individual fitness levels and gout severity.

Water-Based Exercises:

- **Overview:** Exploring the benefits of aqua aerobics and swimming for individuals with gout.

- **Benefits:** Reduced joint stress and enhanced flexibility due to buoyancy.

- **Considerations:** Safety tips for engaging in water-based exercises and recommended routines.

Wearable Technology:

- **Overview:** How fitness trackers and smartwatches can support gout management.

- **Benefits:** Monitoring activity levels, tracking exercise progress, and managing health data.

- **Considerations:** Choosing the right technology and integrating it into your routine effectively.

Emerging Therapies and Technologies

Cryotherapy and Gout:

- **Overview:** The use of cryotherapy (cold therapy) to manage inflammation and pain associated with gout.

- **Benefits:** Potential reduction in swelling and discomfort.

- **Considerations:** Guidelines for safe and effective use of cryotherapy.

Electrical Stimulation:

- **Overview:** Exploring the use of electrical stimulation devices to support muscle recovery and joint function.

- **Benefits:** Enhanced muscle strength and reduced pain.

- **Considerations:** Proper use and consultation with a healthcare provider.

Virtual Reality (VR) Rehabilitation:

- **Overview:** Innovative VR programs designed for rehabilitation and exercise.

- **Benefits:** Engaging and interactive exercise routines tailored to individual needs.

- **Considerations:** Assessing the availability and effectiveness of VR programs for gout management.

Integrating Alternative Therapies
Acupuncture

- **Overview:** The practice of acupuncture as a complementary therapy for managing gout symptoms.

- **Benefits:** Potential reduction in pain and improvement in joint function.

- **Considerations:** Choosing a qualified practitioner and evaluating the effectiveness of acupuncture for your condition.

Massage Therapy

- **Overview:** Using massage techniques to alleviate muscle tension and improve joint mobility.

- **Benefits:** Increased circulation, reduced pain, and enhanced relaxation.

- **Considerations:** Types of massage beneficial for gout sufferers and finding a skilled therapist.

Other Modalities

Chiropractic Care:

- **Overview:** Exploring chiropractic adjustments for managing joint pain and improving function.

- **Benefits:** Potential for enhanced joint alignment and pain relief.

- **Considerations:** Working with a chiropractor experienced in treating gout and understanding the limitations of this therapy.

Herbal Remedies:

- **Overview:** Evaluating the use of herbal supplements and remedies for gout management.

- **Benefits:** Potential anti-inflammatory effects and support for overall health.

- **Considerations:** Consulting with healthcare providers before starting any new supplements and ensuring they do not interfere with conventional treatments.

Evaluating Effectiveness and Safety

Evidence-Based Practice:

- **Overview:** Understanding the importance of using evidence-based approaches when integrating alternative therapies.

- **Benefits:** Ensuring treatments are supported by scientific research and proven to be effective.

- **Considerations:** Staying informed about current research and clinical guidelines.

Monitoring and Adjusting:

- **Overview:** The need for ongoing evaluation of the effectiveness and safety of alternative therapies.

- **Benefits:** Adjusting treatments based on individual responses and changing needs.

- **Considerations:** Keeping track of symptoms and progress, and making necessary modifications to your therapy plan.

Consulting with Healthcare Providers:

- **Overview:** The importance of involving healthcare professionals when exploring advanced and alternative therapies.

  - **Benefits:** Receiving personalized advice and ensuring treatments are safe and appropriate.

  - **Considerations:** Sharing information about all therapies being used and discussing any potential interactions or concerns.

This section provides you with highlighted insights into strategies and techniques for managing gout, emphasizing the importance of staying informed about innovative methods and integrating alternative therapies in a safe and effective manner.

Staying Active for Life

Maintaining Long-Term Motivation

Setting New Goals and Challenges

Reevaluating Fitness Goals:

- **Overview:** Periodically reassessing your fitness goals to stay motivated and aligned with your health needs.

- **Strategies:** Setting incremental milestones and celebrating achievements to maintain enthusiasm.

Incorporating Variety:

- **Overview:** Introducing new types of exercises and activities to keep your routine fresh and engaging.

- **Strategies:** Exploring different fitness classes, sports, or outdoor activities that interest you.

Finding Joy in Physical Activity:

- **Overview:** Emphasizing the importance of enjoying your exercise routine to ensure long-term commitment.

- **Strategies:** Choosing activities that you genuinely like and incorporating social aspects, such as exercising with friends or joining a group.

Staying Active Despite Challenges

Overcoming Obstacles:

- **Overview:** Identifying common barriers to staying active and developing strategies to overcome them.

- **Strategies:** Addressing issues such as time constraints, lack of motivation, or physical limitations with practical solutions.

Adaptive Equipment and Modifications:

- **Overview:** Utilizing adaptive equipment or modifying exercises to accommodate changes in physical condition.

- **Strategies:** Exploring tools and modifications that can make physical activity more accessible and enjoyable.

Adapting to Life Changes

Adjusting Routines as Needed

-Life Transitions:

- **Overview:** Navigating changes such as aging, injury, or illness that may impact your exercise routine.

- **Strategies:** Adjusting your activities and goals to fit new circumstances while maintaining an active lifestyle.

Flexible Routines:

- **Overview:** Creating a flexible exercise plan that can be adapted to different phases of life.

- **Strategies:** Developing a routine that can be easily modified as needed without losing motivation.

Staying Active Through Different Life Stages

Youth and Early Adulthood:

- **Overview:** Focusing on building a strong foundation for lifelong fitness during early life stages.

- **Strategies:** Encouraging regular activity and healthy habits from a young age.

Midlife and Aging:

- **Overview:** Adapting exercise routines to address age-related changes and maintain mobility and strength.

- **Strategies:** Emphasizing exercises that support joint health, balance, and overall well-being in later years.

Managing Chronic Conditions:

- **Overview:** Integrating exercise into the management of other chronic conditions that may arise with age.

- **Strategies:** Collaborating with healthcare providers to ensure exercise plans are safe and effective.

Continuing Education and Advocacy

Staying Informed About Gout Research

Latest Developments:

- **Overview:** Keeping up-to-date with the latest research and advancements in gout management and treatment.

 - **Strategies:** Engaging with credible sources, attending conferences, and participating in online forums.

Educational Resources:

 - **Overview:** Utilizing books, articles, and reputable websites to enhance your knowledge about gout.

 - **Strategies:** Regularly exploring new resources and staying informed about emerging treatments and strategies.

Advocating for Gout Awareness and Support

Raising Awareness:

 - **Overview:** Promoting understanding and recognition of gout within the community and beyond.

- **Strategies:** Participating in awareness campaigns, sharing personal experiences, and supporting research initiatives.

Building Support Networks:

- **Overview:** Connecting with other gout sufferers and healthcare professionals to create a supportive community.

- **Strategies:** Joining support groups, online forums, and local organizations focused on gout advocacy and support.

Getting Involved:

- **Overview:** Engaging in activities that contribute to the broader gout community and support system.

- **Strategies:** Volunteering, fundraising, or participating in events that promote gout awareness and research.

This section provides information to maintaining long-term motivation for staying active, adapting to life changes, and engaging in ongoing education and advocacy efforts. Emphasizing the importance of finding joy in physical activity and staying informed to enhance both personal well-being and community support.

Understanding and Managing Comorbidities

Common Comorbid Conditions with Gout

Overview:

Gout often coexists with other health conditions, creating a complex health profile that requires a multifaceted approach to management. Some of the most common comorbidities include:

- **Hypertension (High Blood Pressure):** Individuals with gout frequently have high blood pressure, which can exacerbate the risk of cardiovascular complications.

- **Diabetes:** There is a strong association between gout and type 2 diabetes, with both conditions sharing common risk factors such as obesity and metabolic syndrome.

- **Cardiovascular Disease:** Gout is linked to an increased risk of heart disease, including coronary artery disease and heart failure.

Strategies:

- **Holistic Management:** Addressing these comorbidities involves a comprehensive approach that targets all aspects of health, including diet, exercise, and medication.

- **Integrated Lifestyle Changes:** Adopting lifestyle changes such as reducing sodium intake for hypertension, monitoring blood sugar levels for diabetes, and following a heart-healthy diet can help manage multiple conditions simultaneously.

- **Regular Monitoring:** Regular health check-ups are crucial for monitoring and managing the interactions between gout and these comorbid conditions.

Exercise Considerations for Comorbid Conditions

Overview:

Exercise plays a vital role in managing comorbid conditions alongside gout. Tailoring exercise recommendations to accommodate these additional health issues ensures that individuals can safely benefit from physical activity.

- **Hypertension:** Exercise can help lower blood pressure and improve cardiovascular health. Low-to-moderate aerobic activities like walking or swimming are recommended.

- **Diabetes:** Regular physical activity helps regulate blood sugar levels and improve insulin sensitivity. Combining aerobic exercises with strength training is beneficial.

- **Cardiovascular Disease:** Engaging in consistent, moderate-intensity exercise can improve heart health and reduce the risk of cardiovascular events.

Strategies:

- **Personalized Exercise Plans:** Work with healthcare providers to develop exercise plans that address specific needs and limitations. For instance, individuals with hypertension should avoid exercises that involve holding the breath (like heavy weightlifting).

- **Gradual Progression:** Start with low-impact exercises and gradually increase intensity based on tolerance and medical advice.

- **Monitoring Health Metrics:** Track key health indicators (e.g., blood pressure, blood sugar levels) to ensure exercise remains safe and effective. Adjust the exercise routine as needed based on these metrics.

Consulting with Specialists

Overview:

Working with healthcare professionals is essential for managing gout and its comorbidities effectively. Specialists can provide tailored advice and coordinate care to address all aspects of health.

- **Rheumatologists:** For gout-specific management, including medication adjustments and managing flare-ups.

- **Cardiologists:** For addressing cardiovascular issues and incorporating heart-healthy practices into exercise routines.

- **Endocrinologists**: For managing diabetes and adjusting treatment plans based on blood sugar levels and overall health.

Strategies:

- **Effective Communication:** Clearly communicate your symptoms, concerns, and goals with specialists. This ensures that all aspects of your health are considered in the treatment plan.

- **Coordinated Care:** Work with all your healthcare providers to create a coordinated care plan that integrates management strategies for gout and its comorbidities.

- **Regular Follow-Ups:** Schedule regular follow-up appointments to monitor progress and make necessary adjustments to your treatment and exercise plans.

By addressing these areas, you can create a comprehensive approach to managing gout alongside other health conditions, improving overall well-being and quality of life.

Psychological Aspects of Chronic Pain

The Impact of Chronic Pain on Mental Health

Overview:

Chronic pain, such as that caused by gout, can have profound effects on mental health. The persistent discomfort and limitations imposed by the condition often lead to psychological challenges, including:

- **Depression:** Chronic pain can lead to feelings of sadness, hopelessness, and a lack of interest in activities once enjoyed. The persistent nature of pain may also contribute to a sense of helplessness or despair.

- **Anxiety:** The unpredictability of gout flare-ups and concerns about future pain episodes can cause significant anxiety. This anxiety may manifest as constant worry, panic attacks, or a generalized sense of unease.

- **Stress and Irritability:** Constant pain can strain the nervous system, leading to heightened stress levels and irritability. This stress can affect relationships, work, and daily functioning.

Strategies:

- **Recognizing Symptoms:** It's crucial to recognize the signs of mental health challenges, such as persistent sadness, changes in sleep or appetite, or excessive worry. Early identification can lead to timely intervention.

- **Seeking Professional Help:** Consulting with mental health professionals, such as therapists or counselors, can provide valuable support and coping strategies. Medication or therapy may be recommended to manage symptoms effectively.

Coping Mechanisms and Stress Management

Overview:

Managing chronic pain requires not only physical care but also mental and emotional resilience. Developing effective coping mechanisms can help mitigate the psychological impact of pain.

Strategies:

- **Mindfulness and Meditation:** Practicing mindfulness helps individuals stay present and reduce the focus on pain. Techniques like deep breathing and guided imagery can help manage stress and promote relaxation.

- **Relaxation Exercises:** Incorporating relaxation exercises such as progressive muscle relaxation or yoga can help reduce muscle tension and promote mental calmness.

- **Therapy Options:** Cognitive-behavioral therapy (CBT) can be particularly effective in changing negative thought patterns and developing coping strategies. Support groups can also provide a sense of community and shared experience.

Building a Resilient Mindset

Overview:

Cultivating a positive and resilient mindset is crucial for coping with chronic pain. A resilient mindset helps individuals navigate the challenges of living with gout, maintaining a hopeful outlook despite setbacks.

Strategies:

- **Positive Affirmations:** Using positive affirmations can help shift focus from pain to strength. Repeating affirmations like "I am strong and capable" or "I can manage my pain" can build mental resilience.

- **Setting Achievable Goals:** Setting small, achievable goals provides a sense of accomplishment and helps maintain motivation. Celebrating these successes, no matter how small, fosters a positive outlook.

- **Engaging in Enjoyable Activities:** Engaging in hobbies and activities that bring joy can distract from pain and boost mood. Whether it's reading, gardening, or spending time with loved ones, these activities can enhance overall well-being.

- **Developing a Support System:** Building a strong support system, including friends, family, and support groups, provides emotional support and encouragement. Sharing experiences and challenges with others who understand can be incredibly empowering.

By addressing the psychological aspects of chronic pain, individuals can better manage the emotional and mental challenges associated with gout. This chapter emphasizes the importance of a holistic approach to health, encompassing both physical and psychological well-being.

Home-Based Exercise Programs

Creating Effective Home Workouts

Overview:

Exercising at home offers flexibility and convenience, making it an excellent option for those managing gout. Home-based workouts can be tailored to individual fitness levels and schedules, helping to maintain an active lifestyle without the need for a gym.

Strategies:

- **Designing Routines:** Start with a warm-up to prepare the body, followed by a balanced mix of aerobic, strength, and flexibility exercises. For example, a routine could include:

- **Low-Impact Aerobic Exercises:** Such as marching in place, dancing, or stepping exercises to elevate heart rate without straining joints.

- **Strength Training:** Using bodyweight exercises like squats, wall push-ups, and leg lifts. If available, light weights or resistance bands can enhance the workout.

- **Flexibility and Stretching:** Incorporate gentle stretching or yoga poses to improve flexibility and reduce muscle tension.

- **Minimal Equipment:** Utilize household items like water bottles for weights or a sturdy chair for support. Investing in basic equipment like resistance bands, a yoga mat, or small dumbbells can enhance workout variety.

Maintaining Motivation for Home Exercise

Overview:

Staying motivated to exercise at home can be challenging due to distractions, limited space, or lack of social interaction. However, with the right strategies, it is possible to maintain a consistent and enjoyable home workout routine.

Strategies:

- **Creating a Dedicated Workout Space:** Designate a specific area in your home for exercise. This space should be free from distractions, well-lit, and comfortable. Having a set space helps mentally prepare for exercise and makes it easier to stick to a routine.

- **Setting Goals:** Establish clear, realistic fitness goals, whether it's improving strength, increasing flexibility, or reducing gout flare-ups. Tracking progress through a journal or app can provide motivation and a sense of accomplishment.

- **Incorporating Variety:** To prevent boredom, vary the types of exercises and routines. Mixing different workouts not only keeps things interesting but also challenges different muscle groups.

- **Using Music and Videos:** Music can be a powerful motivator. Create playlists that energize and uplift you during workouts. Online workout videos can also provide guided sessions and introduce new exercises.

Utilizing Technology for Home Workouts

Overview:

Technology can significantly enhance home-based exercise routines by providing access to a wide range of resources, including instructional videos, fitness apps, and online classes.

Strategies:

- **Fitness Apps:** Utilize apps that offer guided workouts, track progress, and set reminders. Some popular apps cater specifically to those with chronic conditions, providing low-impact exercise options and modifications.

- **Online Classes and Videos:** Platforms like YouTube, fitness websites, and subscription services offer a variety of classes, from yoga and Pilates to strength training and cardio. These resources often cater to different fitness levels and can be followed at your own pace.

- **Virtual Communities:** Joining online fitness communities or social media groups can provide support, encouragement, and accountability. Sharing progress and challenges with others can make the experience more engaging and motivating.

By focusing on home-based exercise programs, this chapter empowers readers to maintain an active lifestyle regardless of access to a gym or outdoor facilities. It emphasizes the importance of creating a conducive environment, setting goals, and leveraging technology to stay motivated and engaged in regular physical activity.

The Role of Family and Social Support

Involving Family in Your Fitness Journey

Overview:

Incorporating family members into your fitness and gout management routine can provide emotional support, increase motivation, and make the journey more enjoyable. Family involvement can also help them better understand your condition and its challenges.

Strategies:

- **Communicating Your Needs:** Openly discuss your goals, limitations, and the importance of staying active with your family. Explain how exercise helps manage gout and improve overall well-being.

- **Shared Activities:** Engage in activities that the whole family can enjoy, such as walking, cycling, or swimming. This not only promotes physical health but also strengthens family bonds.

- **Supportive Roles:** Encourage family members to take on supportive roles, such as joining you for workouts, reminding you to stay active, or preparing healthy meals together. This involvement fosters a shared commitment to health.

Building a Supportive Social Network

Overview:

Having a network of friends and peers who understand and support your journey with gout can be invaluable. Social support can provide encouragement, share experiences, and offer practical advice.

Strategies:

- **Connecting with Others:** Join local or online support groups specifically for gout sufferers or individuals with chronic pain. These communities offer a safe space to share experiences and learn from others facing similar challenges.

- **Maintaining Relationships:** Keep in touch with friends who encourage your healthy lifestyle choices. Share your progress, set shared fitness goals, or simply enjoy social activities that do not trigger gout.

- **Peer Support:** Partner with a friend or acquaintance who also wants to stay active. Having a workout buddy can provide mutual motivation and accountability.

Engaging in Community Activities

Overview:

Participating in community events and groups related to health and wellness can provide additional support and resources. These activities can introduce new fitness opportunities and help you connect with like-minded individuals.

Strategies:

- **Finding Local Groups:** Look for local health and wellness clubs, walking groups, or exercise classes. Community centers, gyms, and health clinics often offer programs tailored to various fitness levels and interests.

- **Attending Health Events:** Participate in community health fairs, seminars, and workshops on gout management, exercise, and nutrition.

These events provide valuable information and the chance to meet health professionals and peers.

- **Volunteering and Advocacy:** Engage in advocacy efforts to raise awareness about gout and chronic pain. Volunteering for related causes can be fulfilling and connect you with others passionate about the same issues.

Make an effort to recognize the importance of involving family and building a supportive social network in managing gout and maintaining an active lifestyle. By fostering strong relationships and engaging with the community, readers can find the motivation and encouragement needed to stay committed to their health journey.

Conclusion

As we come to the end of this guide, let's take a moment to revisit the key concepts and strategies covered in this book. We began by understanding the nature of gout, its causes, symptoms, and how it affects daily life. Recognizing the importance of staying active, we explored the numerous benefits that exercise brings to those living with gout, from reducing inflammation and improving joint function to enhancing mental well-being.

We delved into the specifics of creating a safe and effective exercise routine, tailored to individual needs and fitness levels.

We discussed various types of exercises, including low-impact aerobic activities, strength training, flexibility exercises, and how to incorporate them into a balanced plan.

Additionally, we emphasized the importance of nutrition, hydration, and managing flare-ups, providing practical advice to support long-term health.

We examined the role of psychological resilience, the impact of chronic pain on mental health, and the significance of family and social support. We also looked at advanced strategies, including emerging therapies and innovative exercise methods, and highlighted the value of home-based workouts and community involvement.

Encouragement for Continued Effort

Living with gout presents unique challenges, but it's important to remember that you have the power to make positive changes. The journey toward managing gout and maintaining an active lifestyle is ongoing and requires dedication, patience, and adaptability. By staying informed, seeking support, and continually setting new goals, you can continue to improve your quality of life.

Remember, every step you take towards managing your gout and staying active is a step towards a healthier, more fulfilling life. Celebrate your successes, learn from setbacks, and keep moving forward. Your efforts are a testament to your resilience and determination, and they inspire others who may be facing similar challenges.

As we end this book, I want to leave you with a message of resilience and hope. Living with gout can sometimes feel overwhelming, but remember, every challenge is an opportunity to grow stronger. You have already shown incredible courage by taking steps to learn, adapt, and improve your health. This journey is not just about managing gout; it's about embracing a lifestyle that supports your overall well-being.

Each day brings a new chance to move forward, no matter how small the steps may seem. It's okay to have setbacks or face difficult days— what matters is your commitment to keep going. Embrace the ups and downs as part of your unique journey. Celebrate your progress, however minor it may appear, and recognize the strength you've built along the way.

Staying active and healthy isn't just a goal; it's a continuous process that enriches your life. Whether you're walking, stretching, lifting weights, or simply taking a moment to breathe deeply, each action contributes to your wellness. Surround yourself with supportive people, seek inspiration from others, and keep exploring new ways to enjoy physical activity.

Remember, you are not alone in this journey. There are countless others who understand what you're going through and who are rooting for your success. Together, we can redefine what it means to live with gout—not as a limitation, but as a challenge that we rise to meet with strength, determination, and a positive spirit.

Keep moving, keep growing, and most importantly, keep believing in yourself. Your journey is a testament to your resilience, and it will continue to inspire those around you. Stay active, stay hopeful, and embrace the vibrant, healthy life you deserve.

Cheers...

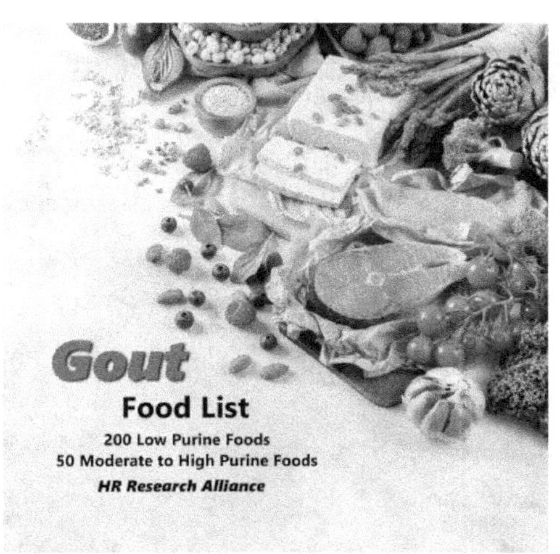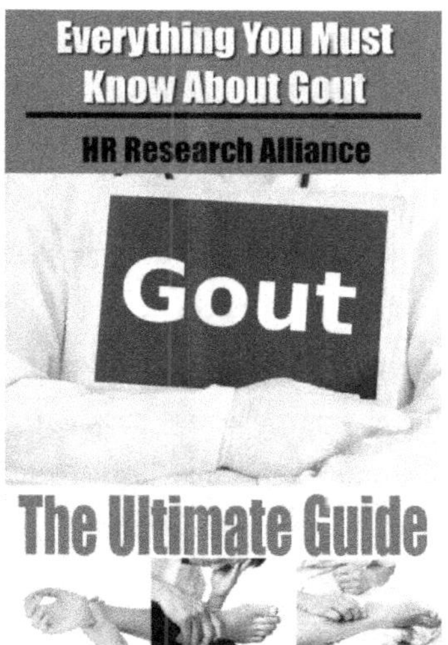

More books on gout that are beneficial to you. You can search for & find these books on the same platform you discovered this guide.

Disclaimer

The information provided in this book is intended for general informational purposes only and is not a substitute for professional medical advice, diagnosis, or treatment. The content is based on personal experiences, research, and expert opinions, but it should not be considered a comprehensive guide for managing gout or any other medical condition.

Readers are strongly encouraged to consult with their healthcare providers before starting any new exercise program, making dietary changes, or using any nutritional supplements. Individual health conditions and needs can vary greatly, and only a qualified healthcare professional can provide personalized advice and treatment.

The author and publisher disclaim any liability for any adverse effects or consequences resulting from the use of the information contained in this book. The exercises, dietary suggestions, and other strategies discussed are meant to support general health and well-being, not to replace medical treatment or advice from a licensed healthcare professional.

Always seek the advice of your physician or other qualified health provider with any questions you may have regarding a medical condition. Here's a suggested

All rights reserved.